DASH DIET COOKBOOK FOR SENIORS

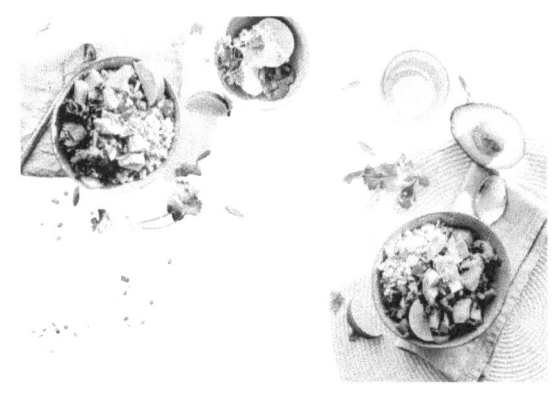

Delicious and Nutritious Recipes Tailored for Senior Health

By

Miranda Montblanc

TABLE OF CONTENTS

INTRODUCTION

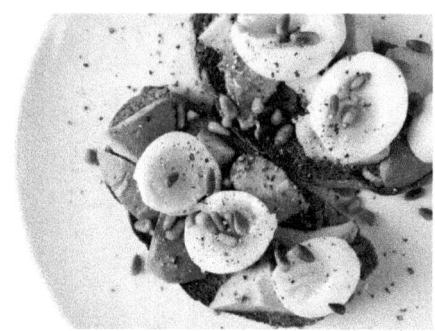

Welcome to the world of healthy living with the DASH (Dietary Approaches to Stop Hypertension) diet, specially crafted for seniors like you. As we age, our nutritional needs change, and it becomes even more vital to adopt a balanced and nourishing diet. The DASH diet, renowned for its effectiveness in lowering high blood pressure and promoting heart health, is not just a diet; it's a lifestyle.

In this cookbook, we have curated a collection of delicious, easy-to-make recipes tailored to meet the dietary requirements of seniors. These recipes are not only tasty but also designed to support your overall well-being. Whether you are a seasoned cook or a novice in the kitchen, these recipes will inspire you to create flavorful meals that are beneficial for your health.

As we embark on this culinary journey together, you will discover a variety of dishes that emphasize fresh, whole foods, lean proteins, and heart-healthy fats. We have incorporated plenty of fruits, vegetables, whole grains, and low-fat dairy products, all of which are essential components of the DASH diet. By following the recipes in this cookbook, you can enjoy flavorful meals while taking care of your heart and overall health.

In addition to the mouthwatering recipes, this cookbook provides valuable tips on grocery shopping, meal planning, and portion control, making it easier for you to maintain a healthy lifestyle. We believe that good nutrition should never compromise on taste, and with the recipes in this book, you can savor every bite while nourishing your body.

So, let's embark on this exciting culinary adventure together, where you can discover the joy of cooking, the pleasure of eating, and the benefits of following the DASH diet for a healthier, happier you. Here's to your well-being and the delightful flavors that await you in the pages that follow. Happy and healthy cooking!

DASH Diet Principles

The DASH (Dietary Approaches to Stop Hypertension) diet focuses on promoting heart health and preventing or controlling hypertension (high blood pressure). Its principles are rooted in a balanced and nutrient-rich eating plan, emphasizing the following key components:

1. _**Fruits and Vegetables**_: The DASH diet encourages a high intake of fruits and vegetables rich in vitamins, minerals, and antioxidants. These foods provide essential nutrients and help lower blood pressure.

2. _**Whole Grains:**_ Whole grains like brown rice, quinoa, and whole wheat bread are high in fiber, which aids in digestion and contributes to a feeling of fullness. They also help regulate blood sugar levels.

3. _**Lean Proteins**_: The diet includes lean protein sources such as poultry, fish, beans, nuts, and low-fat dairy products. These proteins are lower in saturated fat and provide necessary amino acids for body maintenance and repair.

4. _**Low-Fat Dairy:**_ Low-fat or fat-free dairy products are recommended for their calcium content, which supports bone health. They are also lower in saturated fat, reducing the risk of heart disease.

5. _Nuts, Seeds, and Legumes:_ These protein-rich foods are high in fiber and healthy fats, offering a satisfying snack option while contributing to heart health.

6. _Limited Saturated and Trans Fats_: The DASH diet restricts foods high in saturated and trans fats, such as fatty meats, full-fat dairy products, and processed snacks. These fats can raise cholesterol levels and increase the risk of heart disease.

7. _Reduced Sodium Intake:_ Lowering sodium (salt) intake is a central aspect of the DASH diet. By reducing salt, blood pressure can be effectively controlled, reducing the risk of hypertension and related heart problems.

Benefits of the DASH Diet for Seniors

1. _Heart Health_: The DASH diet's emphasis on whole foods and low sodium intake helps seniors maintain a healthy heart, reducing the risk of heart disease and stroke.

2. _Blood Pressure Management_: Seniors are prone to hypertension, which can lead to various health issues. The DASH diet's focus on low-sodium, nutrient-rich foods helps regulate blood pressure, promoting overall cardiovascular health.

3. _Bone Health_: The inclusion of low-fat dairy products in the DASH diet ensures an adequate intake of calcium and vitamin D, supporting bone health and reducing the risk of osteoporosis in seniors.

4. *__Weight Management:__* The diet's focus on whole foods and portion control aids in weight management, which is crucial for seniors to maintain a healthy body weight and reduce the risk of obesity-related diseases.

5. *__Improved Digestion:__* High-fiber foods like fruits, vegetables, and whole grains promote healthy digestion, preventing constipation and promoting a comfortable digestive system for seniors.

6. *__Nutrient-Rich Diet:__* The DASH diet ensures seniors receive essential nutrients, vitamins, and minerals necessary for overall well-being, energy, and vitality, promoting a better quality of life in their golden years.

By following the DASH diet principles, seniors can enjoy these benefits and lead a healthier, more active life, promoting longevity and overall well-being.

Chapter 1

Understanding the DASH Diet

In the realm of senior health and nutrition, the DASH (Dietary Approaches to Stop Hypertension) diet stands as a beacon of balanced eating and heart-conscious choices. Rooted in decades of research, the DASH diet champions a holistic approach to nutrition, emphasizing the consumption of whole foods and mindful portion control.

At its core, the DASH diet revolves around the abundant intake of fruits and vegetables. These colorful, nutrient-packed offerings form the cornerstone of a diet geared towards cardiovascular health. Rich in vitamins, minerals, and antioxidants, fruits and vegetables not only satisfy the palate but also nurture the body, promoting vitality and longevity in seniors.

Whole grains find their place in the DASH diet, offering a hearty dose of fiber and essential nutrients. Brown rice, quinoa, and whole wheat products feature prominently, aiding digestion and regulating blood sugar levels. Lean proteins, sourced from poultry, fish, legumes, and nuts, ensure seniors receive the necessary amino acids without the burden of excess saturated fats. This balanced approach to protein intake supports muscle maintenance and overall body function.

The DASH diet advocates for the inclusion of low-fat dairy products, recognizing their role in bone health. Calcium and vitamin D, found abundantly in these products, strengthen bones and joints, crucial for the aging population. Additionally, the diet discourages the consumption of foods high in saturated and trans fats, steering seniors away from the pitfalls of heart disease and related complications.

Central to the DASH diet's success is the careful management of sodium intake. Seniors, often susceptible to hypertension, benefit immensely from reduced salt consumption. By embracing the flavors of herbs and spices over excessive salt, seniors can safeguard their cardiovascular health, maintaining optimal blood pressure levels.

Beyond its dietary components, the DASH diet champions a lifestyle marked by mindful eating habits. Portion control takes precedence, ensuring seniors derive satisfaction from their meals without overindulging. This conscientious approach fosters a healthy relationship with food, preventing the pitfalls of obesity and related ailments.

In essence, the DASH diet embodies a philosophy that transcends mere sustenance. It encapsulates a way of life, where nutrition becomes a means to holistic well-being. For seniors, this dietary approach paves the way to a future marked by vitality, resilience, and the pleasures of a well-nourished existence. By understanding and embracing the principles of the DASH diet, seniors can embark on a journey towards a healthier, heart-conscious lifestyle, savoring the richness of life in its entirety.

DASH Diet Basics

At its core, the DASH (Dietary Approaches to Stop Hypertension) diet is not just a meal plan; it's a holistic approach to eating that focuses on cultivating heart health and overall well-being. Its fundamental principles revolve around mindful choices and balanced nutrition.

1. *Abundant Fruits and Vegetables*:
The DASH diet places a strong emphasis on incorporating a variety of fruits and vegetables into daily meals. These vibrant, nutrient-dense foods are packed with vitamins, minerals, and antioxidants, promoting optimal health and providing essential energy for daily activities.

2. _Wholesome Whole Grains_:
Whole grains such as brown rice, whole wheat, and oats feature prominently in the DASH diet. These grains are rich in fiber, aiding digestion and providing a sustained release of energy. They also contribute to a feeling of fullness, preventing overeating and supporting weight management.

3. _Lean Proteins:_
Proteins are sourced from lean options like poultry, fish, beans, nuts, and legumes. These protein sources are low in saturated fats, making them heart-friendly. Protein is essential for muscle maintenance and repair, ensuring seniors remain active and agile.

4. _Low-Fat Dairy_:
Low-fat or fat-free dairy products provide necessary calcium and vitamin D for bone health. These dairy options maintain the richness of taste without compromising on nutritional value, promoting strong bones and reducing the risk of osteoporosis.

5. _Healthy Fats_:
The DASH diet encourages the consumption of healthy fats found in sources like avocados, olive oil, and nuts. These fats are beneficial for heart health and overall well-being. They add flavor to meals and contribute to a feeling of satisfaction without the negative effects of saturated fats.

6. _Sodium Moderation_:

One of the key aspects of the DASH diet is limiting sodium intake. By reducing the consumption of salt, seniors can manage blood pressure effectively. Herbs, spices, and natural flavorings are used to enhance taste, ensuring heart health without sacrificing flavor.

7. *Mindful Portion Control:*
The DASH diet emphasizes mindful portion control, preventing overeating and promoting a healthy weight. Seniors are encouraged to savor their meals, paying attention to hunger and fullness cues. This approach fosters a positive relationship with food and prevents unnecessary calorie intake.

By embracing these basic principles, seniors can not only manage their blood pressure but also enjoy a varied and flavorful diet that supports overall health and vitality. The DASH diet serves as a roadmap to a heart-healthy lifestyle, empowering seniors to make conscious choices that nurture their well-being and enhance their quality of life.

Detailed Explanation of Recommended Food Groups

1. *Fruits and Vegetables:*
Fruits and vegetables are nutrient powerhouses, providing essential vitamins, minerals, and antioxidants. Seniors are encouraged to consume a

variety of colorful fruits and vegetables to ensure a wide range of nutrients. Berries, citrus fruits, leafy greens, and cruciferous vegetables are particularly beneficial. These foods are low in calories and high in fiber, promoting digestive health and overall well-being.

2. _Whole Grains:_

Whole grains like brown rice, quinoa, whole wheat pasta, and oats are rich in fiber and complex carbohydrates. They provide sustained energy, regulate blood sugar levels, and support digestive health. Whole grains are also a good source of B vitamins, which are important for energy production and brain health.

3. _Lean Proteins:_

Lean protein sources such as skinless poultry, fish, beans, lentils, tofu, and nuts are essential for seniors. Protein is vital for muscle maintenance, repair, and immune function. These protein sources are low in saturated fats, making them heart-healthy options. Fatty fish like salmon and trout provide omega-3 fatty acids, which are beneficial for heart and brain health.

4. _Low-Fat Dairy:_

Low-fat or fat-free dairy products like milk, yogurt, and cheese are rich in calcium and vitamin D, supporting bone health and preventing osteoporosis. Seniors can choose fortified dairy alternatives like almond milk or soy milk if they are lactose intolerant. These products provide the same nutrients without the lactose content.

5. _Healthy Fats:_

Healthy fats, found in avocados, olive oil, nuts, and seeds, are essential for brain health and hormone regulation. These fats are unsaturated and contribute to a feeling of satiety. Including moderate amounts of these fats in the diet can enhance flavor and provide a sense of satisfaction without compromising heart health.

Portion Control and Balanced Nutrition

Portion control is a fundamental aspect of the DASH diet, ensuring that seniors consume appropriate quantities of food to maintain a healthy weight. It involves being mindful of serving sizes and not overeating, even when consuming nutritious foods. Balanced nutrition, on the other hand, involves consuming a variety of foods in the right proportions to meet the body's nutritional needs.

Seniors can practice portion control by using smaller plates, bowls, and utensils. Eating slowly and savoring each bite can help recognize feelings of fullness, preventing overindulgence. Planning meals and snacks in advance can also aid in portion control, ensuring that seniors have balanced, nutritious options readily available.

Customizing the DASH Diet for Seniors

Customizing the DASH diet for seniors involves considering individual dietary needs, preferences, and health conditions. Seniors may have specific dietary restrictions or medical conditions that require special attention. For instance, individuals with diabetes need to monitor carbohydrate intake, while those with kidney issues may need to limit certain nutrients like potassium and phosphorus.

Customization can also involve adapting recipes to accommodate dietary preferences and ensuring that meals are enjoyable. Seniors can personalize the DASH diet by choosing a variety of foods within each food group, experimenting with herbs and spices for flavor, and incorporating cultural or regional dishes that align with DASH diet principles.

Consulting a healthcare provider or a registered dietitian can be immensely helpful in customizing the DASH diet to meet the specific needs of seniors. These professionals can provide personalized guidance, ensuring that seniors receive optimal nutrition tailored to their individual requirements and preferences.

Adjusting Sodium Intake for Older Adults

As seniors are more susceptible to hypertension and related health issues, adjusting sodium intake becomes crucial. Reducing sodium can help manage blood pressure and promote overall cardiovascular health. Here are some strategies for older adults to adjust their sodium intake:

1. *Read Labels:* Seniors should carefully read food labels to identify high-sodium items and choose low-sodium alternatives. Many processed and packaged foods contain hidden sodium.

2. *Cook at Home*: Home-cooked meals allow seniors to control the amount of salt added to their dishes. Using herbs, spices, lemon juice, and vinegar can enhance flavor without relying on excessive salt.

3. *Limit Processed Foods:* Processed foods like canned soups, sauces, and frozen meals are often high in sodium. Seniors should limit their consumption of these items and opt for fresh, whole foods instead.

4. *Choose Fresh Foods:* Fresh fruits, vegetables, and lean meats are naturally low in sodium. Seniors

should focus on incorporating these items into their diet and minimize the intake of processed foods.

5. _**Use Potassium-Rich Foods**_**:** Potassium helps counterbalance the effects of sodium on blood pressure. Seniors can include potassium-rich foods like bananas, oranges, potatoes, and spinach in their diet.

6. _**Be Mindful at Restaurants:**_ When dining out, seniors can request dishes to be prepared with less salt or ask for sauces and dressings to be served on the side. Restaurant meals often contain hidden sodium, so it's essential to be vigilant.

Incorporating Senior-Friendly Nutrients

As seniors have unique nutritional needs, incorporating specific nutrients into their diet is essential for maintaining good health and vitality. Here are some senior-friendly nutrients to focus on:

1. _**Calcium and Vitamin D**_**:** Essential for bone health, seniors should include low-fat dairy products, fortified plant-based milk, leafy greens, and exposure to sunlight to ensure an adequate intake of calcium and vitamin D.

2. _**Omega-3 Fatty Acids:**_ Found in fatty fish like salmon and walnuts, omega-3 fatty acids support heart health and cognitive function. Seniors can also consider fish oil supplements if recommended by their healthcare provider.

3. _**Fiber**_: Fiber aids in digestion, prevents constipation, and supports a healthy gut. Seniors can get fiber from whole grains, fruits, vegetables, legumes, and nuts.

4. _**B Vitamins**_: B vitamins, especially B12 and folate, are crucial for energy production and brain health. Seniors can find these vitamins in fortified foods, lean meats, eggs, and leafy greens.

5. _**Protein**_: Adequate protein intake is vital for maintaining muscle mass and strength in older adults. Seniors can include lean meats, poultry, fish, eggs, dairy, legumes, and nuts in their diet.

6. _**Antioxidants**_: Found in colorful fruits and vegetables, antioxidants help combat oxidative stress and inflammation. Seniors can enjoy berries, tomatoes, carrots, and bell peppers to incorporate antioxidants into their diet.

By adjusting sodium intake and incorporating these senior-friendly nutrients, older adults can support their overall health, boost their energy levels, and maintain a strong and resilient body as they age. Consulting a healthcare provider or a registered dietitian can provide personalized recommendations tailored to individual needs and health conditions.

Chapter 2

Senior-Specific Health Considerations

As individuals age, specific health considerations become crucial to maintaining overall well-being and quality of life. Here are some key health considerations tailored for seniors:

1. *Regular Health Check-ups:*
   Seniors should schedule regular check-ups with healthcare providers to monitor blood pressure, cholesterol levels, bone density, and other vital indicators. Regular screenings for diabetes, cancer, and eye and dental health are also essential.

2. *Medication Management:*
   Seniors often take multiple medications. It's crucial to manage medications effectively, understanding dosage, interactions, and potential side effects. Regular medication reviews with healthcare providers can help optimize drug regimens.

3. *Nutrition and Hydration:*
   Maintaining a balanced diet rich in nutrients is vital. Seniors should focus on calcium, vitamin D, and protein intake. Hydration is equally important;

seniors may have reduced thirst signals, so they should drink water regularly.

4. _Fall Prevention_:
Falls are a significant concern for seniors. Removing tripping hazards, installing handrails, and ensuring proper lighting at home can prevent falls. Balance and strength exercises can also improve stability.

5. _Mental Health:_
Seniors should pay attention to their mental well-being. Social engagement, hobbies, and cognitive activities can support mental health. Regular social interactions and staying mentally active are crucial for cognitive function.

6. _Vision and Hearing:_
Regular eye and hearing exams are essential. Vision and hearing impairments can impact mobility and overall safety. Corrective measures like glasses or hearing aids can significantly improve quality of life.

7. _Dental Health:_
Oral health is linked to overall health. Regular dental check-ups are important for preventing oral infections and maintaining proper nutrition. Seniors should brush and floss regularly and use mouthwash if recommended by a dentist.

8. _Physical Activity:_
Regular physical activity, tailored to individual abilities, is crucial. It maintains muscle mass, bone

density, and cardiovascular health. Activities like walking, swimming, or gentle yoga can be beneficial.

9. _Sleep_:

Seniors need adequate sleep for overall health and energy. Establishing a regular sleep schedule, creating a relaxing bedtime routine, and ensuring a comfortable sleep environment are important for quality sleep.

10. _Social Connections_:

Maintaining social connections with family, friends, and the community is essential for emotional well-being. Social interactions provide support, reduce feelings of isolation, and contribute to overall happiness.

By addressing these senior-specific health considerations, individuals can lead a fulfilling and healthy life in their golden years. Regular healthcare visits, a balanced lifestyle, and a supportive social network play pivotal roles in ensuring a high quality of life for seniors.

Managing Hypertension and Heart Health

Managing hypertension (high blood pressure) is paramount for heart health, especially in seniors.

Hypertension, if left uncontrolled, can lead to serious cardiovascular issues, making it crucial to adopt lifestyle changes that promote a healthy heart. One such impactful approach is embracing the DASH (Dietary Approaches to Stop Hypertension) diet.

Importance of DASH Diet in Reducing Hypertension

The DASH diet holds significant importance in the realm of managing hypertension due to its focus on heart-healthy foods and balanced nutrition. Here's why the DASH diet is instrumental in reducing hypertension:

1. *Lowering Sodium Intake:*
The DASH diet emphasizes reducing sodium intake, a key factor in hypertension. By limiting salt consumption, blood pressure levels can be effectively controlled, reducing the strain on the heart and arteries.

2. *Rich in Potassium, Magnesium, and Calcium*:
The DASH diet promotes foods high in potassium, magnesium, and calcium. These minerals play a crucial role in regulating blood pressure. Potassium helps balance sodium levels, magnesium relaxes blood vessels, and calcium supports smooth muscle contraction in the heart and blood vessels.

3. *Emphasis on Whole Foods:*

The DASH diet encourages the consumption of whole foods, such as fruits, vegetables, whole grains, lean proteins, and nuts. These foods are naturally low in saturated fats, cholesterol, and sodium, making them heart-healthy choices that contribute to overall cardiovascular well-being.

4. _High in Fiber:_
Fiber-rich foods like fruits, vegetables, whole grains, and legumes are key components of the DASH diet. Dietary fiber aids in digestion, supports weight management, and helps regulate blood sugar levels. Additionally, a high-fiber diet is linked to lower blood pressure.

5. _Balanced Nutritional Profile:_
The DASH diet provides a balanced nutritional profile, ensuring seniors receive essential vitamins, minerals, and antioxidants. This balanced approach supports overall health and vitality, reducing the risk factors associated with hypertension and heart disease.

6. _Long-Term Health Benefits:_
Adopting the DASH diet as a long-term dietary approach not only helps in managing hypertension but also offers a wide array of health benefits. It can aid in weight management, prevent other chronic diseases, and promote overall well-being, allowing seniors to lead an active and fulfilling life.

In conclusion, the DASH diet's emphasis on low sodium intake, potassium-rich foods, whole grains, and balanced nutrition makes it a powerful tool in managing hypertension and promoting heart health. By incorporating DASH diet principles into their daily lives, seniors can take proactive steps towards a healthier heart, reducing the risk of cardiovascular complications and enhancing their overall quality of life.

Heart-Healthy Recipes and Tips

Maintaining heart health is essential, and adopting a heart-healthy diet can significantly contribute to overall cardiovascular well-being. Here are some heart-healthy recipes and tips tailored to support a robust heart:

1. ***Grilled Salmon with Citrus Salsa:***
   - Ingredients:
     - Fresh salmon fillets
     - Olive oil
     - Salt and pepper
     - For Citrus Salsa: Mixed citrus fruits (oranges, grapefruits, and lemons), red onion, cilantro, olive oil, salt, and pepper.
   - **Preparation:**
     - Season salmon fillets with olive oil, salt, and pepper. Grill until cooked through.

- Prepare citrus salsa by mixing chopped citrus fruits, red onion, cilantro, olive oil, salt, and pepper. Serve over grilled salmon.

2. *Quinoa and Vegetable Stir-Fry:*
  - *Ingredients:*
    - Cooked quinoa
    - Assorted vegetables (bell peppers, broccoli, carrots, snow peas)
    - Low-sodium soy sauce
    - Garlic, minced
    - Ginger, grated
    - Olive oil
  - *Preparation*:
    - Sauté minced garlic and grated ginger in olive oil. Add chopped vegetables and stir-fry until tender.
    - Add cooked quinoa and low-sodium soy sauce. Toss everything together until well combined.

3. *Berry and Yogurt Parfait:*
  - *Ingredients*:
    - Mixed berries (strawberries, blueberries, raspberries)
    - Low-fat Greek yogurt
    - Honey or agave syrup
    - Granola (optional)
  - *Preparation*:

- Layer a glass with low-fat Greek yogurt, mixed berries, and a drizzle of honey or agave syrup.
- Repeat the layers. Top with granola for added crunch (optional).

Heart-Healthy Cooking Tips

1. *Use Healthy Fats:* Opt for heart-healthy fats like olive oil, avocados, and nuts. These fats support good cholesterol levels and are beneficial for heart health.

2. *Limit Salt:* Use herbs, spices, and citrus juices to add flavor to dishes instead of excessive salt. High sodium intake can contribute to hypertension.

3. *Include Fiber*: Fiber-rich foods like whole grains, fruits, vegetables, and legumes promote digestive health and can help lower cholesterol levels.

4. *Choose Lean Proteins*: Opt for lean protein sources like poultry, fish, tofu, and legumes. Trim visible fats from meats and remove skin from poultry to reduce saturated fat intake.

5. *Control Portion Sizes*: Be mindful of portion sizes to avoid overeating. Using smaller plates and bowls can help regulate portion control effectively.

6. *Stay Hydrated*: Drink plenty of water throughout the day. Proper hydration supports overall bodily functions, including heart health.

7. *Minimize Processed Foods:* Processed foods are often high in unhealthy fats, sodium, and added

sugars. Limit their consumption and focus on whole, natural foods.

By incorporating these heart-healthy recipes and tips into daily life, individuals can promote heart health, reduce the risk of cardiovascular diseases, and enjoy delicious, nourishing meals that support overall well-being. Remember, a balanced diet, combined with regular physical activity and a healthy lifestyle, forms the foundation for a healthy heart.

Bone Health and Osteoporosis

Understanding Bone Health:
Bone health is vital at every stage of life, but it becomes especially critical as we age. Bones provide structural support to the body, protect internal organs, and act as a reservoir for essential minerals like calcium and phosphorus. To maintain optimal bone health, it's crucial to focus on a balanced diet, regular physical activity, and lifestyle choices that support strong and healthy bones.

Osteoporosis:
Osteoporosis is a condition characterized by weak, brittle bones that are more prone to fractures and breaks. It occurs when the body loses too much bone, makes too little bone, or both. Osteoporosis

often progresses without noticeable symptoms until a fracture occurs, making it a silent but serious health concern, especially among older adults, particularly postmenopausal women.

Factors Affecting Bone Health

Several factors influence bone health, including:

1. *Diet*: Adequate calcium and vitamin D intake are crucial for bone health. Calcium is the building block of bones, while vitamin D helps the body absorb calcium.

2. *Physical Activity:* Weight-bearing exercises and resistance training strengthen bones and improve bone density. Regular physical activity also enhances balance, reducing the risk of falls and fractures.

3. *Lifestyle Choices:* Avoiding smoking and excessive alcohol consumption promotes better bone health. Both smoking and heavy alcohol intake can negatively impact bone density.

4. *Hormones*: Changes in hormone levels, especially in women after menopause, can lead to bone loss. Hormone replacement therapy under medical supervision may be recommended in some cases.

Maintaining Bone Health

1. _**Calcium-Rich Diet**_: Include dairy products, leafy green vegetables, almonds, and fortified foods in your diet to ensure an adequate calcium intake. 2. _**Vitamin D**_: Spend time outdoors in sunlight to enable the body to produce vitamin D naturally. Fatty fish and fortified foods are also good sources of vitamin D. 3. _**Regular Exercise**_: Engage in weight-bearing exercises like walking, jogging, dancing, and resistance training to strengthen bones and improve balance. 4. _**Limit Caffeine and Salt**_: Excessive consumption of caffeine and salt can lead to calcium loss. Moderation is key to maintaining a healthy balance. 5. _**Regular Check-ups**_: Consult a healthcare provider for bone density screenings and advice on supplements if necessary, especially for older adults and postmenopausal women.

By adopting a balanced diet, staying physically active, and making positive lifestyle choices, individuals can promote bone health and reduce the risk of osteoporosis, ensuring a strong and resilient skeletal system well into their later years.

Calcium-Rich Recipes for Strong Bones

Incorporating calcium-rich foods into your diet is essential for maintaining strong bones and preventing osteoporosis. Here are two delicious recipes packed with calcium:

1. _Creamy Spinach and Kale Smoothie:_
  - _Ingredients_:
   - 1 cup fresh spinach leaves
   - 1 cup kale leaves, stems removed
   - 1 ripe banana
   - 1 cup low-fat yogurt or almond milk
   - 1 tablespoon chia seeds (optional)
   - 1 tablespoon honey or maple syrup (optional, for sweetness)
   - Ice cubes (optional)
  - _Instructions_:
   1. In a blender, combine spinach, kale, banana, yogurt or almond milk, chia seeds, and honey or maple syrup.
   2. Blend until smooth and creamy.
   3. Add ice cubes if desired and blend again until the smoothie reaches your desired consistency.
   4. Pour into a glass and enjoy this calcium-packed green smoothie!

2. _Baked Salmon with Lemon and Dill:_

- Ingredients:
   - 2 salmon fillets
   - 1 lemon, thinly sliced
   - 2 tablespoons fresh dill, chopped
   - Salt and black pepper, to taste
   - 1 tablespoon olive oil
 - _Instructions_:
   1. Preheat the oven to 375°F (190°C).
   2. Season the salmon fillets with salt, black pepper, and chopped dill.
   3. Place lemon slices on top of each salmon fillet.
   4. Drizzle olive oil over the salmon.
   5. Bake in the preheated oven for 15-20 minutes or until the salmon is cooked through and flakes easily with a fork.
   6. Serve the baked salmon with your favorite side dishes and enjoy a calcium-rich meal.

These recipes not only provide a rich source of calcium but also offer a delightful culinary experience. Including such calcium-packed dishes in your regular meals can contribute significantly to your bone health and overall well-being.

Tips for Improving Bone Density in Seniors

1. _Calcium-Rich Diet:_

Encourage seniors to consume calcium-rich foods like dairy products, leafy green vegetables, almonds, and fortified foods. Aim for the recommended daily calcium intake to support bone health.

2. _Vitamin D Intake:_

Adequate vitamin D is essential for calcium absorption. Seniors should spend time outdoors to absorb sunlight, consume vitamin D-fortified foods, and consider supplements if advised by a healthcare provider.

3. _Regular Weight-Bearing Exercise:_

Engage in weight-bearing exercises such as walking, jogging, dancing, or strength training. These activities stimulate bone formation, improve bone density, and enhance balance, reducing the risk of falls and fractures.

4. _Balance and Flexibility Exercises:_

Include balance and flexibility exercises like yoga or tai chi in the routine. These exercises improve stability, reducing the likelihood of falls and fractures.

5. _Limit Caffeine and Salt:_

Excessive caffeine and salt can lead to calcium loss. Encourage moderation in the consumption of coffee, tea, and processed foods to maintain a healthy calcium balance.

6. _Quit Smoking and Limit Alcohol:_

Smoking and excessive alcohol consumption can negatively impact bone density. Seniors should quit smoking and limit alcohol intake to support bone health.

7. _Regular Health Check-ups:_

Regular bone density screenings and check-ups with healthcare providers can help assess bone health and determine appropriate interventions or supplements if necessary.

8. _Maintain a Healthy Weight:_

Maintaining a healthy weight through a balanced diet and regular exercise prevents excessive stress on the bones and reduces the risk of fractures.

9. _Adequate Protein Intake:_

Seniors should ensure they are getting enough protein in their diet. Protein supports muscle strength and overall bone health.

10. _Fall Prevention Measures:_

Implement fall prevention measures at home, such as removing tripping hazards, installing handrails, and using non-slip mats. Preventing falls reduces the risk of fractures, especially in seniors with fragile bones.

11. _Consult a Healthcare Provider:_

Seniors should consult their healthcare provider or a registered dietitian for personalized advice on nutrition, supplements, and exercise tailored to their specific needs and health conditions.

By following these tips and adopting a bone-healthy lifestyle, seniors can improve and maintain their bone density, ensuring a strong and resilient skeletal system as they age.

Chapter 3

Meal Planning for Seniors

Meal planning for seniors is a thoughtful and essential process that can significantly impact overall health and well-being. As individuals age, their nutritional needs change, making it vital to focus on balanced, nutrient-rich meals that cater to specific health concerns. Here are key considerations for effective meal planning tailored to seniors:

1. _Varied and Colorful Diet:_
Encourage seniors to embrace a diverse range of foods, especially fruits and vegetables. A colorful plate signifies a variety of nutrients, vitamins, and minerals essential for vitality. Including a spectrum of colors in meals ensures a wide array of health benefits.

2. _Adequate Protein Intake:_
Protein is vital for seniors to maintain muscle mass and support bodily functions. Include sources of lean protein such as poultry, fish, beans, and nuts. Incorporating protein-rich foods in each meal can aid in overall strength and energy levels.

3. _Mindful Portion Control:_

Seniors should focus on portion control to prevent overeating and maintain a healthy weight. Using smaller plates and bowls can help regulate portion sizes, promoting a sense of satisfaction without excessive calorie intake.

4. _Hydration is Key:_
Adequate hydration is often overlooked but is crucial, especially for seniors. Encourage regular water intake throughout the day. Herbal teas, infused water, and low-sodium broths can add variety while keeping seniors hydrated.

5. _Whole Grains for Sustained Energy:_
Whole grains like brown rice, quinoa, and whole wheat provide sustained energy due to their high fiber content. These grains also aid in digestion and regulate blood sugar levels, making them an ideal choice for seniors.

6. _Healthy Fats for Brain Health:_
Incorporate healthy fats from sources like avocados, olive oil, and nuts. These fats support brain health and provide a feeling of satiety, ensuring seniors enjoy their meals while receiving essential nutrients.

7. _Limit Processed Foods:_
Processed foods are often high in sodium, unhealthy fats, and preservatives. Minimize the consumption of packaged snacks, fast food, and sugary beverages. Opt for whole, unprocessed foods to maximize nutritional benefits.

8. _Customizing to Dietary Needs:_
Be mindful of any dietary restrictions or health conditions. Seniors with diabetes, hypertension, or allergies may require specific modifications. Consulting a healthcare provider or a registered dietitian can provide tailored guidance for accommodating these needs.

9. _Social and Enjoyable Dining:_
Eating is not just about nourishment; it's a social and enjoyable activity. Encourage seniors to share meals with friends or family members. Creating a pleasant dining environment can enhance the overall mealtime experience, promoting better appetite and digestion.

In summary, meal planning for seniors should focus on a well-balanced, colorful diet, mindful portion control, and hydration. Customization based on individual needs and a focus on enjoyable dining experiences are equally important. By following these principles, seniors can enjoy delicious, nutritious meals that support their health and well-being in their golden years.

Nutrition-Packed Meal Ideas

Creating meals that are not only delicious but also packed with nutrients is essential for overall health and well-being. Here are some nutrition-packed meal ideas that incorporate a variety of vitamins, minerals, and essential nutrients:

1. _**Grilled Chicken Salad:**_
  - Grilled chicken breast slices seasoned with herbs and spices.
  - Mixed greens (spinach, kale, arugula) for a variety of vitamins and minerals.
  - Cherry tomatoes and cucumber for hydration and antioxidants.
  - Avocado slices for healthy fats.
  - Nuts or seeds (such as almonds or pumpkin seeds) for added protein and crunch.
  - Dress with olive oil, lemon juice, and a dash of balsamic vinegar.

2. _**Quinoa and Vegetable Stir-Fry:**_
  - Cooked quinoa for a protein and fiber boost.
  - Colorful bell peppers, broccoli, carrots, and snow peas for vitamins and antioxidants.
  - Tofu or tempeh for plant-based protein.
  - Light soy sauce, garlic, and ginger for flavor.
  - Garnish with chopped green onions and sesame seeds.

3. _**Salmon and Vegetable Foil Packets:**_
  - Salmon fillet for omega-3 fatty acids and protein.

- Asparagus, zucchini, and bell peppers for vitamins and fiber.
- Drizzle with olive oil, sprinkle with your favorite herbs and spices.
- Seal ingredients in foil packets and bake for a flavorful and nutritious meal.

4. _Mediterranean Chickpea Bowl:_
- Cooked chickpeas for plant-based protein and fiber.
- Chopped cucumbers, tomatoes, and red onions for freshness and vitamins.
- Kalamata olives and feta cheese for flavor.
- Drizzle with olive oil, lemon juice, and sprinkle with oregano.
- Serve over a bed of whole grain rice or quinoa.

5. _Vegetable and Lentil Soup:_
- Lentils for protein and fiber.
- Mixed vegetables like carrots, celery, tomatoes, and spinach for vitamins and minerals.
- Low-sodium vegetable broth for the base.
- Herbs and spices like turmeric, cumin, and bay leaves for flavor.
- Serve hot with a side of whole grain bread for a filling and nutritious meal.

These meal ideas provide a balance of carbohydrates, proteins, healthy fats, vitamins, and minerals. Customizing them with seasonal produce and herbs can enhance flavors and nutritional content, ensuring a well-rounded and nourishing diet.

Sample Meal Plans

Breakfast
1. Option 1:
   - Greek yogurt parfait with layers of low-fat Greek yogurt, mixed berries, and granola.
   - Whole grain toast with avocado spread.
   - Green tea or herbal tea.
2. Option 2:
   - Vegetable omelette with spinach, tomatoes, and mushrooms.
   - Whole grain toast or multigrain muffin.
   - Fresh orange juice or a piece of whole fruit.

Lunch:
1. Option 1:
   - Grilled chicken salad with mixed greens, cherry tomatoes, cucumbers, and avocado.
   - Quinoa or brown rice on the side.
   - Olive oil and lemon dressing.
   - A small bowl of mixed berries for dessert.
2. Option 2:
   - Lentil and vegetable soup.
   - Whole grain bread or a small whole grain roll.

- Side salad with mixed greens, chickpeas, and a light vinaigrette.
- Fresh fruit salad for dessert.

Dinner:
1. Option 1:
   - Baked salmon with lemon and dill.
   - Steamed asparagus and quinoa.
   - Mixed green salad with a variety of colorful vegetables.
   - A small serving of dark chocolate for dessert.
2. Option 2:
   - Grilled tofu with teriyaki sauce.
   - Stir-fried broccoli, bell peppers, and carrots.
   - Brown rice or whole grain noodles.
   - Sliced melon or a fruit salad for dessert.

<u>Snacks</u>:
1. Option 1:
   - Handful of mixed nuts (like almonds and walnuts).
   - Low-fat yogurt with honey and a sprinkle of chia seeds.
   - Baby carrots and cucumber slices with hummus dip.
2. Option 2:
   - Fresh fruit, such as an apple or a banana.
   - Whole grain crackers with low-fat cheese.

- Herbal tea or a small smoothie made with spinach, banana, and almond milk.

Remember to stay hydrated throughout the day, opting for water, herbal teas, or infused water with slices of fruits or cucumbers. These sample meal plans provide a variety of nutrients, including proteins, whole grains, fruits, vegetables, and healthy fats, ensuring a well-balanced and satisfying diet. Adjust portion sizes and food choices based on individual dietary needs and preferences.

Nutritional benefits of each suggested meal

Breakfast:
1. *__Greek Yogurt Parfait:__*
   - *__Benefits:__* Rich in protein and probiotics, Greek yogurt supports digestion and promotes a feeling of fullness. Berries provide antioxidants and essential vitamins, while granola offers fiber and complex carbohydrates for sustained energy.
2. *__Vegetable Omelette:__*
   - *__Benefits__*: Eggs are a good source of high-quality protein. Spinach, tomatoes, and mushrooms provide vitamins, minerals, and antioxidants. Whole grain toast adds fiber and carbohydrates for energy.

Lunch:
1. *Grilled Chicken Salad:*
      - *Benefits*: Grilled chicken is a lean protein source. Mixed greens offer vitamins A and K, along with fiber. Avocado provides healthy fats, and quinoa or brown rice offers complex carbohydrates and additional protein.
2. *Lentil and Vegetable Soup:*
      - *Benefits*: Lentils are rich in fiber and protein. Vegetables add vitamins and minerals. Whole grain bread provides carbohydrates, and the side salad offers additional nutrients and fiber.

Dinner:
1. *Baked Salmon with Lemon and Dill:*
      - *Benefits*: Salmon is a fatty fish rich in omega-3 fatty acids, supporting heart and brain health. Asparagus provides vitamins A and C, while quinoa offers protein and fiber. Mixed greens in the salad add vitamins and minerals.
2. *Grilled Tofu with Teriyaki Sauce:*
      - *Benefits*: Tofu is a plant-based protein source. Broccoli, bell peppers, and carrots offer vitamins, fiber, and antioxidants. Brown rice or whole grain noodles provide complex carbohydrates for energy.

Snacks:
1. *Mixed Nuts:*

    - _Benefits_: Nuts are a source of healthy fats, protein, and various vitamins and minerals. They provide sustained energy and support heart health.

2. _Fresh Fruit:_

    - _Benefits_: Fruits like apples, bananas, and melons provide vitamins, minerals, and fiber. They are naturally sweet and offer a quick energy boost.

3. _Low-Fat Yogurt with Chia Seeds:_

    - _Benefits_: Yogurt contains probiotics for gut health, and chia seeds offer omega-3 fatty acids and fiber, promoting fullness and supporting digestion.

4. _Whole Grain Crackers with Cheese:_

    - Benefits: Whole grain crackers provide fiber and carbohydrates, while low-fat cheese offers protein and calcium, supporting bone health.

These meals are designed to provide a balanced mix of macronutrients (proteins, carbohydrates, and fats) and micronutrients (vitamins and minerals), ensuring overall nourishment and promoting optimal health and well-being.

Adapting Portion Sizes

Adapting portion sizes is essential for seniors to maintain a healthy weight, support energy levels, and ensure overall well-being. As metabolism slows down with age, portion control becomes even more crucial. Here are some guidelines for appropriate portion sizes tailored for seniors:

1. *Listen to Hunger and Fullness Cues:*
Encourage seniors to eat mindfully, paying attention to their body's hunger and fullness signals. Stop eating when comfortably satisfied, even if there's food left on the plate.

2. *Balance Nutrients:*
Ensure meals consist of a balance of proteins, carbohydrates, healthy fats, and plenty of vegetables. A balanced diet provides essential nutrients and supports overall health.

3. *Use Smaller Plates and Bowls:*
Opt for smaller plates and bowls. Smaller dishware gives the illusion of larger portions, making the meal feel satisfying without overeating.

4. *Avoid Second Helpings:*
Discourage second servings, especially at restaurants or social gatherings. Encourage seniors to wait for a few minutes before deciding if they are still hungry.

5. *Include a Variety of Foods:*
A diverse diet ensures a range of nutrients. Encourage seniors to incorporate different foods, textures, and colors into their meals. Variety also makes meals more enjoyable and satisfying.

6. *Practice Portion Distortion:*

Educate seniors about portion distortion, where large restaurant servings can influence perceptions of a standard portion size. Encourage sharing entrees at restaurants or opting for smaller-sized portions if available.

7. *Measure and Divide Foods:*

Use measuring cups or a food scale to understand appropriate portion sizes for different foods. Pre-portioning snacks into small containers can prevent overeating.

8. *Prioritize Nutrient-Dense Foods:*

Emphasize nutrient-dense foods like fruits, vegetables, whole grains, lean proteins, and healthy fats. These foods offer more nutrients per calorie, making them ideal choices for seniors.

9. *Be Mindful of Liquid Calories*:

Beverages like sugary drinks, alcohol, and high-calorie coffee beverages can add significant calories. Encourage water, herbal tea, and other low-calorie beverages for hydration.

10. *Monitor Condiments and Sauces:*

Condiments and sauces can add extra calories and sodium. Use them sparingly and opt for healthier alternatives like herbs, spices, and lemon juice for flavor.

By following these guidelines, seniors can adapt portion sizes to meet their nutritional needs without overindulging. This approach supports overall health, energy levels, and a healthy weight, promoting a balanced and satisfying diet.

Avoiding Overeating and Maintaining a Healthy Weight

Maintaining a healthy weight is essential for overall well-being and reducing the risk of chronic diseases. Here are some strategies to avoid overeating and support weight management, especially tailored for seniors:

1. *Eat Mindfully*:
Pay attention to physical hunger and fullness cues. Eat slowly, savoring each bite, and pause between bites. This helps the body recognize fullness, preventing overeating.

2. *Portion Control:*
Use smaller plates, bowls, and utensils to control portion sizes. Avoid second servings, and be mindful of portion distortion, especially in restaurants where servings tend to be larger.

3. *Plan Balanced Meals:*
Prioritize balanced meals with a mix of lean proteins, whole grains, plenty of vegetables, and healthy fats. Balanced meals provide essential nutrients, promote satiety, and prevent excessive snacking.

4. *Stay Hydrated:*

Drink water throughout the day. Sometimes, feelings of hunger are actually signs of dehydration. Drinking water before meals can also help control appetite.

5. _Include Fiber-Rich Foods:_

Fiber-rich foods like fruits, vegetables, whole grains, and legumes promote fullness and aid digestion. They keep you feeling satisfied longer, reducing the likelihood of overeating.

6. _Mindful Snacking:_

Choose healthy snacks like fresh fruits, nuts, or yogurt. Portion snacks into small containers to avoid mindlessly eating from large packages. Be mindful of portion sizes even during snack times.

7. _Identify Emotional Eating Triggers:_

Be aware of emotional triggers that lead to overeating, such as stress, boredom, or loneliness. Find alternative ways to cope with emotions, such as exercise, hobbies, or talking to friends and family.

8. _Practice Regular Physical Activity:_

Engage in regular physical activity tailored to individual abilities. Exercise not only burns calories but also helps regulate appetite and improves overall well-being.

9. _Avoid Highly Processed Foods:_

Processed foods often contain excessive calories, unhealthy fats, and sugars. Limit intake of fast food, sugary snacks, and sugary beverages, as they contribute to weight gain.

10. _Seek Support:_

Don't hesitate to seek support from healthcare providers, nutritionists, or support groups if struggling with overeating or weight management. Professional guidance can provide personalized strategies and motivation.

By incorporating these practices into daily life, seniors can avoid overeating, maintain a healthy weight, and promote overall health and well-being. Adopting a balanced diet, staying physically active, and being mindful of portion sizes are key steps toward a healthier lifestyle.

Chapter 4

Easy and Delicious DASH Diet Recipes

1. DASH Diet Veggie Stir-Fry:
Ingredients:
- 1 tablespoon olive oil
- 1 onion, thinly sliced
- 2 cloves garlic, minced
- 1 bell pepper, thinly sliced
- 1 zucchini, sliced
- 1 cup broccoli florets
- 1 cup sliced mushrooms
- 1 can (15 oz) low-sodium chickpeas, drained and rinsed
- 2 tablespoons low-sodium soy sauce
- 1 teaspoon honey or agave syrup
- 1 teaspoon grated fresh ginger
- 2 green onions, chopped (for garnish)
- Cooked brown rice or quinoa (optional, for serving)

Instructions:
1. In a large skillet, heat olive oil over medium heat. Add onions and garlic, and sauté until fragrant.

2. Add bell pepper, zucchini, broccoli, and mushrooms to the skillet. Stir-fry the vegetables until they are tender-crisp.

3. Add chickpeas to the skillet and stir to combine.

4. In a small bowl, whisk together soy sauce, honey, and grated ginger. Pour the sauce over the vegetable mixture and toss to coat evenly.

5. Cook for a few more minutes until the vegetables are cooked to your desired tenderness.

6. Garnish with chopped green onions.

7. Serve the stir-fry over cooked brown rice or quinoa if desired.

2. DASH Diet Berry Parfait

Ingredients:

- 1 cup low-fat Greek yogurt
- 1 cup mixed berries (strawberries, blueberries, raspberries)
- 2 tablespoons honey or maple syrup
- 1/4 cup granola
- Fresh mint leaves (for garnish)

Instructions:

1. In a bowl, mix the Greek yogurt with honey or maple syrup until well combined.

2. In serving glasses or bowls, layer the yogurt mixture with mixed berries.

3. Repeat the layers until the glasses are filled.

4. Top each parfait with a sprinkle of granola for added crunch.

5. Garnish with fresh mint leaves.

6. Refrigerate for a few hours or enjoy immediately.

These recipes are not only easy to prepare but also delicious and in line with the DASH diet principles. They are packed with nutrients, low in sodium, and feature a variety of colorful vegetables and fruits, making them a healthy choice for anyone following the DASH diet.

Breakfast Delights

1. *Berry Banana Smoothie Bowl:*
Ingredients:
- 1 frozen banana
- 1 cup mixed berries (strawberries, blueberries, raspberries)
- 1/2 cup low-fat Greek yogurt
- 1 tablespoon honey or agave syrup
- Toppings: sliced fresh fruits, granola, chia seeds, shredded coconut, and a drizzle of honey
Instructions:
1. In a blender, combine the frozen banana, mixed berries, Greek yogurt, and honey. Blend until smooth and creamy.
2. Pour the smoothie into a bowl.
3. Top with sliced fresh fruits, granola, chia seeds, shredded coconut, and a drizzle of honey.

4. Enjoy this nutritious and visually appealing smoothie bowl for a delightful breakfast experience.

2. *Avocado Toast with Poached Egg:*
***Ingredients*:**
- 1 slice of whole grain bread, toasted
- 1/2 ripe avocado, mashed
- 1 poached egg
- Salt, pepper, and red pepper flakes (to taste)
- Fresh herbs (such as cilantro or chives) for garnish
- Optional: a squeeze of lemon juice

***Instructions*:**
1. Spread the mashed avocado evenly over the toasted whole grain bread.
2. Carefully place the poached egg on top of the avocado.
3. Season with salt, pepper, and red pepper flakes to taste.
4. Garnish with fresh herbs and, if desired, a squeeze of lemon juice for added freshness.
5. Enjoy your delicious and nutrient-packed avocado toast with a perfectly poached egg.

These breakfast delights not only taste great but also provide a good balance of carbohydrates, healthy fats, proteins, and essential vitamins and minerals to fuel your morning. Customize them with your favorite toppings and flavors for a delightful breakfast experience.

Nutritious and easy-to-make breakfast recipes

1. *Greek Yogurt Parfait:*
Ingredients:
- 1 cup low-fat Greek yogurt
- 1/2 cup granola
- 1/2 cup mixed fresh berries (such as strawberries, blueberries, raspberries)
- 1 tablespoon honey or maple syrup
- Optional: a sprinkle of chia seeds or sliced almonds
Instructions:
1. In a glass or bowl, layer half of the Greek yogurt at the bottom.
2. Add a layer of mixed berries on top of the yogurt.
3. Sprinkle a layer of granola over the berries.
4. Drizzle half of the honey or maple syrup over the granola.
5. Repeat the layers with the remaining yogurt, berries, granola, and honey or maple syrup.
6. Optionally, top the parfait with a sprinkle of chia seeds or sliced almonds for added texture and nutrition.
7. Enjoy your delicious and nutritious Greek yogurt parfait!

2. *Avocado and Egg Breakfast Wrap:*
Ingredients:

- 1 whole wheat or multigrain wrap or tortilla
- 1/2 ripe avocado, sliced
- 2 eggs, scrambled or fried
- Handful of baby spinach leaves
- Salt, pepper, and a pinch of chili flakes (optional)
- Salsa or hot sauce (optional, for added flavor)

Instructions:

1. Warm the whole wheat or multigrain wrap in a skillet or microwave according to the package instructions.
2. Layer the sliced avocado, scrambled or fried eggs, and baby spinach leaves in the center of the wrap.
3. Season with salt, pepper, and a pinch of chili flakes if desired.
4. Drizzle with salsa or hot sauce for added flavor and a bit of heat.
5. Fold the sides of the wrap over the filling to create a breakfast burrito.
6. Serve warm and enjoy your nutritious and satisfying avocado and egg breakfast wrap!

These breakfast recipes are not only packed with nutrients but also quick to prepare, making them ideal choices for a healthy and hassle-free morning meal. Feel free to customize the ingredients to suit your taste preferences and dietary needs.

Healthy salads, soups, and sandwiches tailored for seniors

Here are some healthy and flavorful lunchtime favorites tailored for seniors:

1. _Grilled Chicken Salad with Berry Vinaigrette_:
Ingredients:
- Grilled chicken breast slices
- Mixed salad greens (spinach, arugula, and romaine lettuce)
- Fresh berries (strawberries, blueberries, raspberries)
- Sliced cucumbers and cherry tomatoes
- Feta cheese, crumbled
- Chopped nuts (such as almonds or walnuts)
- Berry vinaigrette dressing (mix olive oil, balsamic vinegar, a touch of honey, and blended fresh berries)
Instructions:
1. Arrange the grilled chicken slices on a bed of mixed salad greens.
2. Add fresh berries, sliced cucumbers, and cherry tomatoes.
3. Sprinkle crumbled feta cheese and chopped nuts over the salad.
4. Drizzle the berry vinaigrette dressing over the top.
5. Toss gently to combine and enjoy your refreshing and nutritious grilled chicken salad.

2. *Minestrone Soup:*
Ingredients:
- Low-sodium vegetable or chicken broth
- Mixed vegetables (carrots, celery, zucchini, tomatoes)
- Cooked whole grain pasta or brown rice
- Cooked or canned beans (such as kidney beans or chickpeas)
- Fresh basil and oregano (or dried Italian seasoning)
- Salt, pepper, and a splash of olive oil

Instructions:
1. In a large pot, sauté mixed vegetables in a splash of olive oil until slightly softened.
2. Add low-sodium broth and bring to a boil.
3. Reduce heat and add cooked whole grain pasta or brown rice and cooked or canned beans.
4. Season with fresh basil, oregano, salt, and pepper.
5. Simmer until all the ingredients are well combined and flavors meld together.
6. Serve hot and enjoy your hearty and comforting minestrone soup.

3. *Turkey and Avocado Sandwich with Whole Grain Bread:*
Ingredients:
- Sliced turkey breast
- Ripe avocado, mashed

- Whole grain bread slices
- Lettuce leaves, tomato slices, and red onion rings
- Dijon mustard or honey mustard sauce

Instructions:

1. Spread mashed avocado on one slice of whole grain bread.
2. Layer sliced turkey breast, lettuce leaves, tomato slices, and red onion rings.
3. Spread Dijon mustard or honey mustard sauce on the other slice of bread.
4. Put the sandwich together and cut into halves or quarters.
5. Enjoy your wholesome and tasty turkey and avocado sandwich.

These lunchtime favorites are rich in nutrients, balanced in flavors, and easy to prepare, making them ideal choices for seniors looking for healthy and satisfying meals.

Dinner Time Treasures: Flavorful and Balanced Dinner Recipes

1. *Baked Salmon with Roasted Vegetables*:
Ingredients:
- Salmon fillets
- Mixed vegetables (such as broccoli, carrots, and bell peppers)

- Olive oil, lemon juice, garlic powder, salt, and pepper
- Fresh herbs (such as parsley or dill) for garnish
Instructions:
1. Preheat the oven to 375°F (190°C).
2. Place salmon fillets on a baking sheet lined with parchment paper.
3. In a bowl, toss mixed vegetables with olive oil, lemon juice, garlic powder, salt, and pepper.
4. Spread the vegetables around the salmon on the baking sheet.
5. Bake in the preheated oven for 15-20 minutes or until the salmon is cooked through and flakes easily with a fork.
6. Garnish with fresh herbs and serve your flavorful baked salmon with roasted vegetables.

2. *Quinoa and Vegetable Stir-Fry:*
Ingredients:
- Cooked quinoa
- Mixed vegetables (such as bell peppers, broccoli, and snap peas)
- Tofu or chicken breast, cubed
- Low-sodium soy sauce, garlic, and ginger
- Green onions and sesame seeds for garnish
Instructions:
1. In a large skillet or wok, sauté cubed tofu or chicken until cooked through. Remove from the pan and set aside.

2. In the same pan, stir-fry mixed vegetables with garlic and ginger until tender-crisp.
3. Add cooked quinoa and the cooked tofu or chicken back to the pan.
4. Drizzle with low-sodium soy sauce and toss until well combined.
5. Garnish with chopped green onions and sesame seeds before serving.

One-Pot Meals for Convenience

1. _Chicken and Vegetable Brown Rice Casserole:_
Ingredients:
- Chicken thighs or breasts
- Brown rice
- Mixed vegetables (such as carrots, peas, and corn)
- Low-sodium chicken broth
- Garlic, onion, salt, and pepper
- Fresh parsley for garnish
Instructions:
1. In a large pot or casserole dish, combine chicken, brown rice, mixed vegetables, minced garlic, chopped onion, salt, and pepper.
2. Pour in low-sodium chicken broth to cover the ingredients.
3. Cover and simmer over low heat until the chicken is cooked through, rice is tender, and vegetables are soft.

4. Garnish with fresh parsley before serving your comforting one-pot meal.

Snacks and Treats

1. *Yogurt-Dipped Frozen Berries:*
*Ingredients***:**
- Fresh berries (such as strawberries and blueberries)
- Low-fat Greek yogurt
- Honey or maple syrup (optional)
Instructions:
1. Dip fresh berries into low-fat Greek yogurt, covering them completely.
2. Place the yogurt-covered berries on a parchment-lined tray.
3. Freeze until the yogurt hardens, creating a frozen treat.
4. Optional: Drizzle with honey or maple syrup before freezing for added sweetness.

2. *Dark Chocolate-Covered Almonds:*
*Ingredients***:**
- Raw almonds
- Dark chocolate chips (70% cocoa or higher)
Instructions:
1. Melt dark chocolate chips in a microwave-safe bowl in 30-second intervals, stirring until smooth.

2. Dip raw almonds into the melted chocolate, coating them partially.
3. Place the chocolate-covered almonds on a parchment-lined tray.
4. Let them cool and harden in the refrigerator before serving your indulgent yet nutritious snack.

These recipes offer flavorful, balanced dinners and convenient one-pot meals for simplicity. Additionally, the snacks and treats provide healthier alternatives for satisfying your sweet cravings. Enjoy these delicious options tailored for your dining pleasure!

Chapter 5

Practical Tips and Tricks

1. _Stay Hydrated:_
- Keep a water bottle handy to remind yourself to drink water regularly throughout the day.
- Set reminders on your phone or use apps to track your daily water intake.

2. _Meal Preparation:_
- Plan your meals for the week to ensure balanced nutrition.
- Use portion control containers or a food scale to manage serving sizes.

3. _Smart Shopping:_
- Prepare a shopping list before going to the grocery store to avoid impulse purchases.
- Opt for fresh produce, lean proteins, whole grains, and low-fat dairy products.

4. _physical Activity:_
- Engage in activities you enjoy, such as walking, swimming, or gardening, to stay active.
- Consider joining exercise classes or groups specifically designed for seniors.

5. _Safety First:_
- Ensure your home is well-lit and free of clutter to prevent falls.
- Use non-slip mats in the bathroom and kitchen to enhance safety.

6. _Mindful Eating:_
- Eat slowly and savor each bite, appreciating the flavors and textures of your food.
- Avoid distractions like TV or smartphones during meals to focus on eating mindfully.

7. _Social Connections:_
- Stay socially active by joining clubs, volunteering, or spending time with friends and family.
- Plan regular social outings to maintain a strong support network.

8. _Mental Stimulation:_
- Engage in activities that challenge your brain, such as puzzles, reading, or learning new skills.
- Consider taking classes or workshops to stimulate your mind and stay mentally sharp.

9. _Regular Health Check-ups:_
- Schedule regular check-ups with healthcare providers to monitor your health and discuss any concerns.

- Keep track of your medications, and consult your doctor if you experience any side effects.

10. _Quality Sleep:_
- Maintain a regular sleep schedule and create a relaxing bedtime routine.
- Ensure your bedroom is comfortable and conducive to sleep, with a comfortable mattress and minimal noise.

11. _Relaxation Techniques:_
- Practice relaxation techniques such as deep breathing, meditation, or yoga to manage stress.
- Consider hobbies like painting, knitting, or gardening as creative outlets for relaxation.

12. _Digital Literacy:_
- Stay connected with loved ones through social media or video calls to combat feelings of isolation.
- Learn basic digital skills if you're not familiar with technology to stay connected with the digital world.

By incorporating these practical tips and tricks into your daily routine, you can enhance your overall well-being and lead a fulfilling and healthy life in your senior years.

Smart Grocery Shopping for DASH-Friendly Ingredients

When following the DASH (Dietary Approaches to Stop Hypertension) diet, smart grocery shopping plays a crucial role in maintaining a healthy and balanced diet. Here are some tips for choosing DASH-friendly ingredients while grocery shopping:

1. *Focus on Fresh Produce:*
   - Load up your cart with a variety of fresh fruits and vegetables, such as berries, oranges, spinach, kale, broccoli, and bell peppers. These are rich in vitamins, minerals, and antioxidants, and are fundamental to the DASH diet.

2. *Choose Lean Proteins:*
   - Opt for lean protein sources like skinless poultry, fish, tofu, beans, and legumes. These proteins are low in saturated fat and support heart health.

3. *Whole Grains are Key:*
   - Stock up on whole grains such as brown rice, quinoa, whole wheat pasta, oats, and whole grain bread. Whole grains are high in fiber and provide sustained energy.

4. *Low-Fat Dairy and Dairy Alternatives:*
   - Choose low-fat or fat-free dairy products like yogurt, milk, and cheese. For non-dairy options, select almond milk, soy milk, or oat milk fortified with calcium and vitamin D.

5. _Healthy Fats:_

- Incorporate sources of healthy fats, such as avocados, nuts (like almonds and walnuts), seeds (flaxseeds, chia seeds), and olive oil. These fats are heart-friendly and provide essential nutrients.

6. _Mindful Meat Choices:_

- If you consume red meat, choose lean cuts and trim visible fats. Consider poultry and fish as more frequent protein choices.

7. _Canned and Frozen Options:_

- Opt for low-sodium canned goods (like beans and tomatoes) and frozen vegetables without added sauces. These are convenient and can be stored for longer periods.

8. _Read Nutrition Labels:_

- Pay attention to nutrition labels. Look for low-sodium or no-added-salt options, especially in canned soups, sauces, and processed foods. Also, check for added sugars and unhealthy fats.

9. _Limit Processed Foods:_

- Minimize the purchase of processed foods, which often contain high levels of sodium, sugar, and unhealthy fats. Focus on whole, unprocessed foods.

10. _Plan Your Meals:_

- Plan your meals and create a shopping list accordingly. Having a list helps you stick to healthier choices and prevents impulse buys of unhealthy foods.

11. _Stay Hydrated:_
   - Don't forget to include beverages in your grocery list. Choose water, herbal teas, and low-sodium vegetable juices over sugary drinks and high-calorie beverages.

By making thoughtful choices and being mindful of the nutritional content of the foods you buy, you can create a DASH-friendly grocery list that promotes heart health, lowers blood pressure, and supports overall well-being.

Reading Food Labels for Sodium Content

When following the DASH diet, it's crucial to monitor your sodium intake. Here are tips for reading food labels to assess sodium content:

1. _Check the Serving Size:_
   - Start by looking at the serving size to understand how much of the product you'll be consuming.

2. _Look for Sodium Content:_
   - Check the "Sodium" line in the Nutrition Facts panel. Foods with 5% Daily Value (DV) or less of sodium are considered low, while those with 20% DV or more are high in sodium.

3. _Compare Similar Products:_

- Compare sodium content among different brands or versions of the same product. Choose the one with lower sodium content.

4. ___Be Cautious with Processed Foods:___
   - Processed foods like canned soups, sauces, and snacks often contain high sodium. Opt for low-sodium or no-added-salt versions whenever possible.

5. ___Watch for Portion Size___
   - If you plan to eat more than the standard serving size, adjust the sodium content accordingly. For example, if you eat double the serving, you'll consume double the sodium.

Meal Prepping for Seniors

1. ___Plan Balanced Meals:___
   - Plan meals that include a variety of vegetables, lean proteins, whole grains, and healthy fats. Consider colorful vegetables and fruits for added nutrients.

2. ___Use Herbs and Spices:___
   - Enhance flavors without adding sodium by using herbs (such as basil, thyme) and spices (like turmeric, cumin) in your recipes.

3. ___Cook in Batches:___
   - Prepare meals in batches and freeze them in portion-sized containers. This makes it convenient to have healthy, homemade meals on hand.

4. *Choose Low-Sodium Ingredients:*
   - Opt for low-sodium versions of canned goods and condiments. Rinsing canned vegetables and beans can also reduce sodium content.

5. *Mindful Seasoning:*
   - Experiment with vinegar, lemon juice, and low-sodium soy sauce for seasoning. They add flavor without excess sodium.

6. *Include Whole Grains:*
   - Use whole grains like brown rice, quinoa, and whole grain pasta. They're nutritious and provide a good base for various dishes.

7. *Limit Processed Meats*:
   - Minimize processed meats like bacon, sausages, and deli meats. They tend to be high in sodium and unhealthy fats.

8. *Stay Hydrated:*
   - Prepare low-sodium beverages like infused water with fruits and herbs. Staying hydrated is essential for overall health.

By following these tips, you can effectively read food labels to monitor sodium content and prepare nutritious, low-sodium meals, promoting better health and well-being for seniors.

Batch Cooking and Storing Meals for Convenience

1. _Plan Your Meals:_
   - Plan a weekly menu to determine which meals can be batch-cooked. Focus on recipes that freeze well and maintain their texture and flavor after reheating.

2. _Invest in Freezer-Safe Containers:_
   - Use high-quality, freezer-safe containers to store your batch-cooked meals. Consider using individual or portion-sized containers for easy serving.

3. _Label and Date:_
   - Label each container with the meal name and date of preparation. This helps you keep track of the freshness of your meals.

4. _Properly Cool Before Freezing:_
   - Allow hot foods to cool to room temperature before placing them in the freezer. Rapid cooling can help preserve the texture and taste of the food.

5. _Use the Right Method:_
   - Reheat frozen meals in the oven or on the stovetop for more even heating. Microwave meals in short intervals, stirring between, to prevent uneven heating.

6. _Add Moisture if Needed:_
   - If a meal seems dry after reheating, add a splash of water, broth, or sauce to restore moisture and prevent it from becoming too dry.

7. _Avoid Overcooking:_
- Be cautious not to overheat meals, especially those with proteins like chicken or fish, to prevent them from becoming tough or rubbery.

Staying Hydrated and Energized

1. _Drink Water Regularly:_
- Keep a water bottle nearby and take sips throughout the day. Dehydration can lead to fatigue, so staying hydrated is essential.

2. _Incorporate Hydrating Foods:_
- Consume fruits and vegetables with high water content, such as watermelon, cucumber, oranges, and celery, to stay hydrated.

3. _Limit Caffeine and Sugary Drinks_:
- While a moderate amount of caffeine can provide energy, excessive consumption can lead to dehydration. Avoid sugary drinks as they can cause energy crashes.

4. _Balanced Meals and Snacks:_
- Opt for balanced meals and snacks that include a mix of carbohydrates, proteins, and healthy fats. This balance provides sustained energy throughout the day.

5. _Regular Physical Activity:_
- Engage in regular physical activity, even if it's a short walk. Exercise can boost energy levels and overall well-being.

6. _Adequate Sleep:_
- Ensure you're getting enough sleep. Quality rest is crucial for maintaining energy levels and overall health.

By incorporating these practices, you can efficiently batch cook, store meals, reheat food without compromising quality, and stay hydrated and energized throughout the day, promoting a healthy and convenient lifestyle.

Importance of Hydration for Seniors

Hydration is crucial for seniors for several reasons:

1. _Preventing Dehydration:_ Seniors are more prone to dehydration due to changes in their body's water balance, reduced kidney function, and diminished thirst sensation. Proper hydration prevents dehydration-related complications.

2. _Maintaining Cognitive Function_: Adequate hydration supports brain function, memory, and concentration. Dehydration can impair cognitive abilities and lead to confusion and mood changes.

3. _Supporting Physical Health_: Proper hydration helps maintain joint lubrication, regulating body temperature, and supporting cardiovascular health. It also aids in digestion and nutrient absorption.

4. _**Preventing Falls:**_ Dehydration can weaken muscles and lead to dizziness or fainting, increasing the risk of falls. Staying hydrated promotes stability and reduces the risk of accidents.

5. _**Boosting Immune System**_: Hydration supports the immune system by facilitating the movement of immune cells throughout the body, helping the body fight infections and illnesses.

Hydrating and Energizing Drink Recipes

1. _**Citrus Infused Water:**_
**Ingredients**:
- 1 lemon, thinly sliced
- 1 lime, thinly sliced
- 1 orange, thinly sliced
- Fresh mint leaves
- Ice cubes
- Water

**Instructions**
1. Place lemon, lime, and orange slices in a pitcher.
2. Add fresh mint leaves and ice cubes.
3. Fill the pitcher with water and refrigerate for a couple of hours to allow the flavors to infuse.
4. Enjoy this refreshing citrus-infused water.

2. _**Green Tea and Berry Smoothie**_:
**Ingredients**:

- 1 cup brewed green tea, cooled
- 1/2 cup mixed berries (strawberries, blueberries, raspberries)
- 1 tablespoon honey or agave syrup
- 1/2 cup low-fat Greek yogurt
- Ice cubes

Instructions:
1. In a blender, combine brewed green tea, mixed berries, honey or agave syrup, low-fat Greek yogurt, and ice cubes.
2. Blend until smooth and creamy.
3. Pour into a glass and enjoy this antioxidant-rich green tea and berry smoothie.

3. *Coconut Water and Pineapple Energizer:*
Ingredients:
- 1 cup coconut water
- 1/2 cup fresh pineapple chunks
- 1 tablespoon chia seeds (optional)
- 1 teaspoon honey or maple syrup
- Ice cubes

Instructions:
1. In a blender, combine coconut water, fresh pineapple chunks, chia seeds (if using), honey or maple syrup, and ice cubes.
2. Blend until well combined.
3. Pour into a glass and savor this hydrating coconut water and pineapple energizer.

These hydrating and energizing drink recipes are packed with essential nutrients and are perfect for seniors to maintain proper hydration and boost energy levels throughout the day.

CONCLUSION

In the golden years of life, embracing a healthier lifestyle becomes not just a choice, but a gift to oneself. Seniors, like everyone else, deserve to live their lives to the fullest, enjoying every moment with vitality and joy. By adopting healthier habits, staying hydrated, and nourishing the body with wholesome foods, seniors can unlock the door to a life filled with wellness and contentment.

Encouragement and Motivation

Seniors, your journey towards a healthier lifestyle is a testament to your resilience and strength. Each step you take, each nutritious meal you enjoy, and every moment of physical activity you engage in is a celebration of your vitality. Remember, it's never too late to embrace positive changes. Every healthy choice you make is a step toward a more vibrant and fulfilling life.

Surround yourself with positivity, lean on the support of loved ones, and celebrate your progress, no matter how small it may seem. Stay motivated by focusing on the joys of improved health, increased energy, and the ability to savor life's simple pleasures. You are capable of achieving great things, and your well-being is worth every effort.

Embrace each day with enthusiasm, relish the nourishing meals you enjoy, and take pride in the active lifestyle you lead. Your journey towards a healthier you is an inspiration to others and a testament to your resilience. Here's to a future filled with vitality, wellness, and the joy of living life to the fullest!

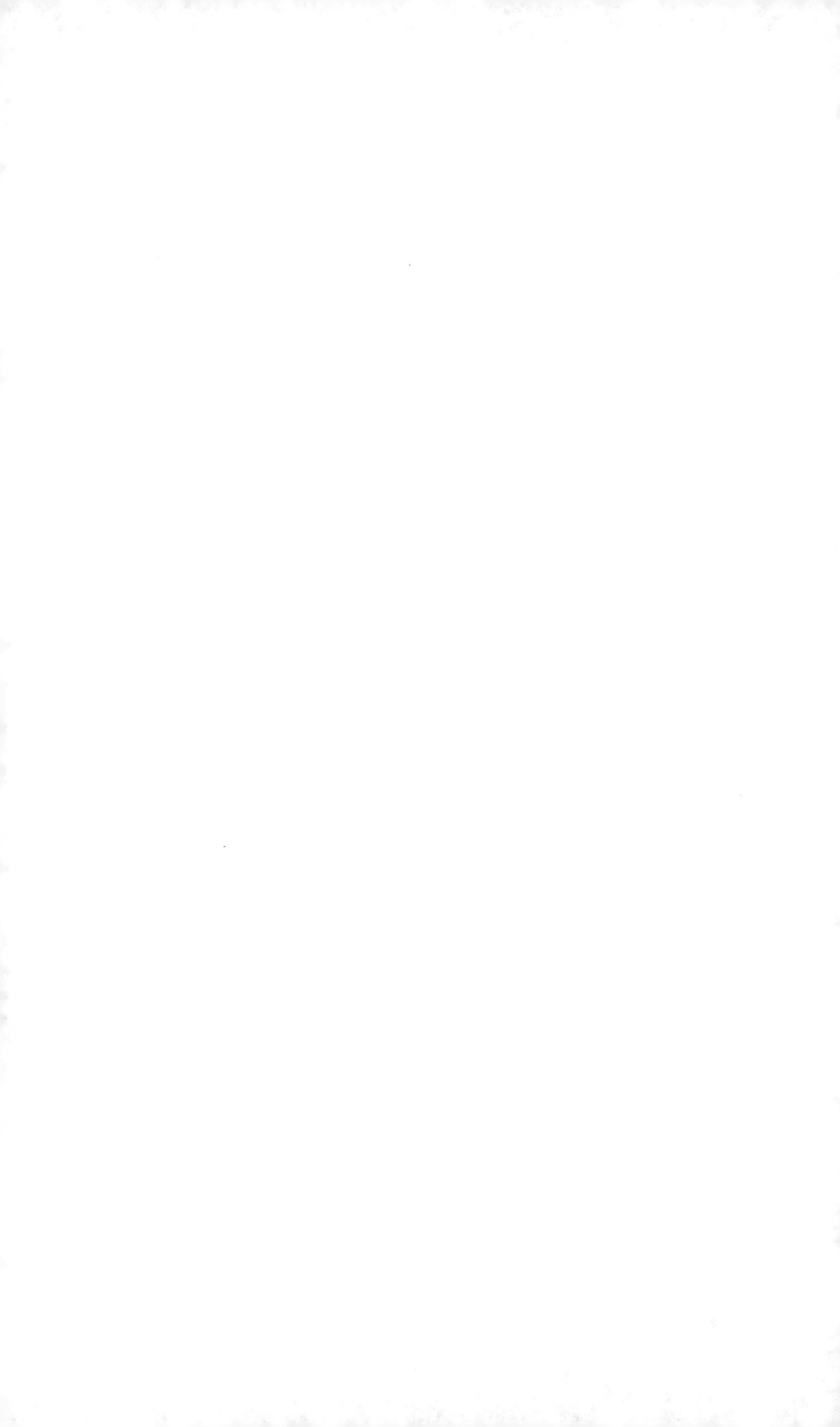